I0412429

Weight Training For Dumbbells
A Guide to Your First Year in the Gym

Disclosure

This e-book is meant to be used for informational purposes only. This book is not meant to be used in substitute for medical treatment or as an alternative to medical advice. Always speak with a health care professional before starting new physical activities to ensure it is safe to do so. Do not use this book for disease prevention or treatment. The reader agrees to use the information in this e-book at his/her own risk and at his/her own choice.

First Printing: 2016

ISBN: 9781520590370

Liam McEachen
979 Parkhill Drive
Parkhill, Ontario N0M 2K0

https://www.youtube.com/channel/UCJIzPmsbgD7V8rjYJHrP65Q

Contents

Introduction 3

Part 1 Your Diet and Nutritional Information 5

Part 2 Supplements and More 24

Part 3 Time to Hit The Gym 36

Part 4 Getting Ready For Your Workout 58

Part 5 Workout Spreadsheets and Game Plan 71

Conclusion 88

Introduction

Have you ever been in the gym and felt a little lost? Have you ever tried to lose weight and ended up doing hours of cardio only to see no results? Have you ever tried to build muscle but didn't know what exercises to do or which supplements to take?

Well you're not alone. We've all been at that point in our lives because everyone is a beginner when they first embark on their fitness journey. I can't even begin to account for all of the wasted time and money that I've spent on workout programs that don't work and supplements that I didn't need.

Over my 8 years of training, I'll be the first to admit, that I didn't do things the smart way. I was never consistent in the gym. I didn't track any of my workouts and I constantly hopped on the biggest supplement buzz to try to build muscle. I have made many mistakes so that you don't have to.

In this e-book I will be telling you about the mistakes I've made in the past and give you the tools for you to reach your goals in the fastest way possible. I will give you the basics of what you need to know, as well as blow away the fog of commercialism so that you can cut the crust off the commercial turd sandwich and reach your goals efficiently. I have put forward many of the concepts that beginners struggle with, or don't know about, and will give you basic information that is understandable and relatable.

My goal is to educate you in a way that will help you to simply see what you need to do to be successful in the gym. This book is for everyone, but will be most beneficial to those of you who have been on your fitness journey for less than a year. So make sure to use the video links disbursed throughout the book (which link to my YouTube channel) and let's get this party started!

Have Fun,

Liam McEachen, B.Bus.

Part 1 Your Diet and Nutritional Information

What Happens When We Workout?

When we do muscle training we are creating small tears in our muscles which our body fixes and rebuilds bigger every time we workout. The old saying, "Whatever doesn't kill you, makes you stronger" is true when it comes to weightlifting. After every workout our body repairs itself and makes itself stronger and bigger.

To start things off, ask yourself this important question: Do you want to lose fat or gain muscle?

Losing Fat

It is not efficient for you to try to lose fat and gain muscle at the same time. Your body doesn't function optimally that way. To lose fat you have to burn more calories than you eat in a day. Your body burns calories through natural processes such as digesting food, as well as doing physical activities, such as running or lifting weights. To find out how many calories your body uses in a day just type in, "Calorie Calculator" into an online search engine. There are many of them and they are very easy to use. This will show you how many calories you need to consume in order to maintain your current body weight. This is also called your maintenance level. From here, in order to lose weight you must either eat less in calories than the number the calorie counter showed you or you must burn calories through physical activity to get you below your maintenance level. You can also do both of these together to help you out even more.

Here is a link to the online calorie calculator that I use: http://www.calculator.net/calorie-calculator.html

For example: Let's say that to maintain your current body weight you need 2500 calories per day. If you want to lose weight you will need to eat less than 2500 calories in a day. I recommend eating no more than 500 calories less than your maintenance level per day because if you do, this will cause your body undue stress and it will be harder for you to lose weight in the long run. This means that you will have only consumed 2000 calories in a day so your body needs another 500 calories to properly function. Where does your body get those 500 calories? Your body will burn fat to compensate for the deficit.

Now let's not forget that we can also lose weight by doing physical activity. If you eat 2500 calories and go for a jog that burns 150 calories you can subtract that 150 from the 2500 calories that you ate which leaves you with 2350 calories that your body can use to operate. This means that your body will, once again, have to burn fat in order to maintain itself so you will be losing fat again!

These two methods can also be used in conjunction with each other. For example, you could eat 2100 in calories throughout the day and also go for run that burns 100 calories and this will leave you with 2000 calories that your body can use to maintain itself. This means that you are in a 500 caloric deficit and your body will burn fat to make up for these missing calories.

The calories you consume have the same value as the calories you burn. Say, if you go over your daily caloric needs and eat 2600 calories throughout the day. Don't worry you can still save yourself! If you do a physical activity that burns 300 calories in total that will bring the calories your body has to use down to 2300 calories, which is still a 200 calorie deficit! Good job!

Gaining Muscle

The bad news is that to gain muscle you will have to gain a bit of fat as well. The good news is you will be gaining muscle! Let's look back to the example for losing weight above. Remember that our maintenance level for our body weight is 2500 calories per day. To gain muscle optimally it is the exact opposite practice. You need to eat more than 2500 calories per day and introduce weight training in order to gain muscle. You will also need to limit cardio as this burns calories needed to build muscle, or you will need to increase your calorie consumption on the days you do cardio. I recommend eating 300-500 calories above your daily caloric maintenance level in order to build muscle as a starting point. It is possible to build a little bit of muscle while you're in a caloric deficit, but you will see much larger muscle gains if you are in a caloric surplus. Therefore it makes more sense to be in a surplus when attempting to gain muscle.

Pro Tip: Define Your Goals and Stick to Them
This felt like an appropriate tip to slip in here because the earlier you make a plan, the sooner you will be successful. Decide on a target weight that you want to get to and work towards that goal until you reach it. When you reach your goal, stop and evaluate your situation and then set a new goal. Whether it be losing weight, gaining weight, or a specific weightlifting goal, just set it!

Be sure to write your goals down as well. A Harvard study suggested that students that had well written out and defined goals were much more likely to be successful in life than those who did not write down their goals. Be sure to review your goal regularly, if not daily, to keep yourself motivated. If you do this, you will not regret it.

One quick note that I want to mention is to make sure you do not have conflicting goals. Remember that the best way to build muscle is to be in a caloric surplus. If your goal is to lose fat and build muscle, that goal is conflicted as it is very difficult to lose fat and build muscle at the same time.

Stick to your goals until you reach them. You don't want to be losing weight one week and gaining weight the next week. If you do this you will be stuck in the same spot because you aren't giving your body the time it needs to make big changes before you start to go in the opposite direction.

Water

According to some sources your body is made up of approximately 60% water. Water helps with kidney function, normalizing bowel function, joint function, regulating temperature, just to name a few. Your muscles consist of a large amount of water which help them to function properly. It is very important to stay hydrated at all times as dehydration can lead to decreased athletic performance. Drinking enough water can allow us to workout longer, fatigue slower, and recover faster.

There are many differing opinions as to how much water you should drink. The old saying was that drinking 8 glasses of water a day is what a person should aim for. This was more of a suggestion and was not based on scientific fact. A quick rule of thumb would be to drink half of your body weight in ounces of water a day. So for a 160lbs person 80oz of water a day should be sufficient. It is also important to note that you can also get water from water dense fruits and vegetables such as apples, pears, oranges, lettuce, tomatoes, celery, and peppers.

Water is used as a lubricant in your body. It helps your whole body run smoothly and function properly. It's such an important part of your diet and you need to be aware of how much you are drinking because it will help you in your workouts.

When Should I Eat My Meals?
There is a lot of speculation as to how many meals one should have in a day and when to eat them. The classical method is to eat 6-8 meals a day and have your calories spread throughout the day. In my personal experience I find this method to be very time consuming. Recent studies are beginning to show that this method of meal timing doesn't provide any real benefit. I was always left hungry after a meal. But there's good news: It doesn't have to be this way!

Personally, I like to feel full after I eat, even if that means going hungry for a period of time beforehand so that I can eat a bigger meal. The good news is that it doesn't matter how many meals you eat as long as you are eating! All things being equal, the amount of meals you have throughout a day won't affect how much muscle you are going to build. For example, a person eating 7 meals a day is still consuming the same amount of calories as a person eating 3 larger meals a day. As long as you are eating the same amount of calories it doesn't matter how many meals you have in a day. With that being said, it may be a little hard on your system if your body has to try to metabolize 3000 calories from one meal in a day. Stick to something that fits into your schedule and will be easiest for you.

There are a few things to know about the timing of meals. This is specifically in regards to the timing of your meals and your workout. A rookie mistake is to eat a big turkey dinner 10 minutes before you are leaving to go to the gym. If you do this, you are going to have a bad workout. Your body uses energy to metabolize food and if you're heading to the gym with a full turkey in your belly, your body is going to be using valuable energy to digest that food that you could be using in your workout. Try to stay away from eating large meals within an hour of your workout and you should be fine.

It is, however, important to not go to the gym when you haven't eaten all day. You will not be able to perform to your full potential because your body will lack the energy it needs to complete your workout. Carbohydrates are key in providing you with the energy you need to get you through your workout. If you don't have any carbs in your system, your body will have to draw from other less efficient sources of energy, such as fat, to help you through your workout. You and your workout will suffer if you go to the gym on an empty stomach so try to avoid this at all costs.

Many sources stress that it is very important to have protein right after your workout. For me, I'm a little more lenient when it comes to this principle because a lot of the time I don't want to be eating a large meal immediately after a hard workout. I try to eat a high protein meal within 2 hours of hitting the gym and this has worked well for me. It gives me the time to be flexible and still provide my body with the nutrients it needs. Again you need to find what works best for you and your body because everyone is different.

Counting Macros.

Counting macros is key to muscle building success, but what is a macro? Macro is short for "macronutrients". Macronutrients consist of proteins, carbohydrates, and fats. Technically speaking, alcohol is a 4th macronutrient, but it is best to try to stay away from alcohol and I will touch on this later. We will be counting macros instead of calories because we need to more accurately track the amount of proteins, carbohydrates, and fats that we are consuming. Calories are made up of macros and the breakdown is as follows:

1 gram of fat = 9 calories

1 gram of carbohydrates = 4 calories

1 gram of protein = 4 calories

For example if we had 100 grams of chicken breast, the macronutrient/caloric breakdown would be as follows:

Fat =   3.6 grams (3.6 grams x 9 calories per 1 gram of fat = 32.4 calories)

Carbohydrates =	0 grams (0 grams x 4 calories per 1 gram of carbohydrates = 0 calories)
Protein =	31 grams (31 grams x 4 calories per 1 gram of protein = 124 calories)
Total Calories =	156.4 calories per 100 grams of chicken breast

If we add the calorics together it comes out to 156.4 calories for 100 grams of chicken. It is so important to know where our calories are coming from rather than to reach a set caloric goal for the day by eating whatever you want.

What do Fats, Carbs, and Proteins do and Where do They Come From?

Fats

Our bodies need fats to function properly and stay healthy. Fats help with hormone regulation, as well as brain function and vitamin absorption. They come mostly from meats, nuts, oils, and fish just to name a few sources. There are three types of fats: Unsaturated fats, saturated fats, and trans fats.

Unsaturated fats are in a liquid state at room temperature. Unsaturated fats are considered to be "good" fats as they help to improve blood cholesterol levels, stabilize heart rhythms, and ease inflammation. There are two types: monounsaturated fats and polyunsaturated fats. Monounsaturated fats come from foods like avocados and olive oil. Polyunsaturated fats come from foods like fish and flax seeds.

Saturated fats are found mostly in animal products such as cheese, chicken, and beef. The old conception used to be that saturated fats caused heart disease. However, recent studies have suggested that saturated fats do not contribute to the risk of heart disease.

Trans fats are made by converting unsaturated fats into a solid state which helps to reduce the chance of the fats spoiling. This process increases the shelf life of the products that have trans fats. Trans fats are also found naturally in small amounts in beef and dairy products. Some health concerns caused by the consumption of trans fats include raising bad LDL cholesterol and lowering good HDL cholesterol, creating inflammation, and increased risk for coronary heart disease. It is best to limit your intake of trans fats as much as possible.

Carbohydrates

There are two ways that our body uses carbohydrates. Our body uses carbohydrates as fuel by burning them when they are consumed or by converting the carbohydrates to glycogen and storing them to be consumed later. Glycogen is stored in the brain, blood, liver, and muscles. The best sources for carbohydrates are fruits, vegetables, and grains. Other sources include pop, candy etc.

Items with a high sugar content aren't necessarily a good source for carbohydrates. For example, pop has a high sugar content and is not a good source of carbs as it is entirely simple sugar. Items with a high level of simple sugar content are not beneficial for you because your body can break them down so quickly that if you don't immediately need to use them as fuel they are converted and stored as fat for future energy use.

Carbohydrates can be simple sugars or complex carbohydrates. Simple sugar simply means that the sugar is only made up of one or two sugar units which the body can quickly and easily break down. A complex carbohydrate contains many different sugar units which takes the body longer to break down and releases energy to your body at a slower pace.

Protein

Protein helps to repair the small tears in your muscles that you get while working out and to prevent muscle loss if you are in a caloric deficit. Meat, fish, egg whites, and protein shakes are good sources of protein.

The Breakdown

The next question to be answered is how much of each macro should I eat in a day? Here is a simple breakdown that you can use to see how much of each macro you should be eating in a day to build muscle:

> Start with Protein: 1 - 1.4 grams of protein per pound of bodyweight. If you are 170lbs you should consume approximately 170 grams of protein per day.

> Fat: 20% of the amount of calories consumed.

> Carbohydrates: Remainder of allotted calories.

Based on a 2200 calorie diet for a person who is 5'10" tall, who exercises 3-5 times per week weighing 170lbs the breakdown would be:

680 calories in protein (170 grams of protein (1 gram per pound)*4 calories)

440 calories in fat (2200 daily caloric intake *20%)

1080 calories in carbohydrates (2200 calories – 680 protein calories – 440 fat calories = 1080 calories from carbohydrates).

Now that we know how many calories of each macro we need to consume, we have to break it down further into how many grams a day that we need so that we can track more accurately.

Fats: 440 calories / 9 calories per gram = 49 grams of fat per day

Carbohydrates: 1080 calories / 4 calories per gram = 270 grams of carbohydrates per day

Protein: 680 calories / 4 calories per gram = 170 grams of protein per day

This person on the 2000 calorie diet would want to eat as close as possible to 49 grams of fat, 270 grams of carbs, and 170 grams of protein per day. It doesn't have to be perfect, but try your best to get as close to the numbers as possible. This will allow you to optimally build muscle because you will have the proper diet in place.

Be sure to adjust your macros as you gain or lose weight. For example, if you gain 10lbs by counting macros, your maintenance level is going to be higher because your body needs more calories to function. It is the opposite if you lose 10lbs, your maintenance level will be lower. Make sure to adjust your macros according to how much you weigh. Personally I would adjust my macros with every 10lb difference in weight.

How Do I Find Out The Amount of Macronutrients In My Food?

This is an easy question to answer, but one that may seem daunting to someone who has never counted macros before. Firstly, you need to buy a scale that measures in grams. A scale is going to be one of the most important tools in your arsenal when it comes to building muscle. Accuracy is key and a scale that measures in grams is part of your golden ticket to success. The second thing you need to do is to check the nutritional label on the food you are eating. This will have a breakdown in grams of the amount of fats, carbs, and protein in the food you are eating. If you are eating less than the full portion on the label make sure you weigh it out on your scale. Let's say that you are eating 100 grams of cereal, but the nutritional information on the package is based on a 200 gram serving size. What do you do? You're screwed! Not actually though, this is an easy fix. All you need to do is divide the weight of the portion you are eating by the serving size on the package. This will give you a percentage. Next you will multiply the listed amounts of grams of fats, carbs, and proteins on the package by the percentage you calculated.

For example, if you are eating 100 grams of cereal with a listed serving size of 200 grams and the macronutrient breakdown on the package is:

Fats – 5 grams per 200 gram serving

Carbs – 80 grams per 200 gram serving

Proteins – 10 grams per 200 gram serving

We would take the 100 gram portion and divide it by the 200 gram listed serving size on the package. This would give us a percentage of 50% (100/200=50%). Next we would multiply the grams of fats, carbs, and proteins listed on the package by 50% to get the amount of grams we will be consuming.

Fats – 5 grams listed * 50% = 2.5 grams consumed

Carbs – 80 grams listed * 50% = 40 grams consumed

Proteins – 10 grams listed * 50% = 5 grams consumed

If you are eating a type of food that doesn't come with nutritional information you can search "calorie counter" on the internet to look up the caloric content of what you are eating. What you want to do is the same process as above by weighing your food and recording your information.

Many fast food places have their menus online with nutritional information. These aren't going to be perfect, but they will be close enough for our purposes. I am not encouraging you to eat fast food unless it's completely unavoidable, but I did want to give you this information so that you know it's available.

Restaurants are a different story. There are many dishes or meals we can't even begin to guess the cooking processes or the amount of ingredients put into making the meal. This makes it next to impossible to accurately track. For example, what type of oil were your vegetables cooked in and how much butter was put on your toast? These are questions that we are not able to answer. My best advice to you is to try to make your own meals as much as possible until you get a good feel for counting macros, just so you are as accurate as possible. I can't even begin to count the amount of times where I've gone out to eat for dinner and went to go weigh myself the next morning to find out I weighed an extra half a pound more than I should have. This was because the amount of food and calories that I thought I was eating were less than what I actually consumed. It's a dangerous road eating out because you never know exactly what you are getting.

If It Fits Your Macros

If It Fits Your Macros or IIFYM is the idea that you can eat whatever types of food you want as long as it fits into your macronutrient breakdown for the day. This idea states that it is ok to stray away from the typical body builder diet of chicken, rice, and broccoli and add variety to your diet. I am a big fan of IIFYM, but there are certain limitations that need to be put in place in order to make IIFYM effective. It is important to understand that being able to eat whatever you want as long as it fits your macros isn't necessarily the best choice. For example, filling your carbohydrate needs for the day by eating a bunch of candy is not conducive to living a healthy lifestyle. Another example would be eating deep fried foods. All though they may fit into your macros, these types of foods have other obvious negative health impacts. If these are types of foods that you love, I would suggest that you continue to eat them, but do so in moderation. Try to limit the amount of these foods in your diet so that you can still enjoy them, but on a much smaller scale.

IIFYM is great because it opens up so many different options to the people who employ this idea. What isn't great is when the user of this idea gets out of hand and they start to lean towards foods that can be harmful to them, but believe they are making good decisions because it "fits their macros." Sticking to whole foods, or foods that don't undergo processing, for the majority of your diet will help to give your body the tools it needs to rebuild itself stronger after every workout.

Alcohol

Alcohol is one of those things in bodybuilding that can give you grief. It's definitely fun to go out with friends and blow off some steam but it is, however, important to understand what we are putting into our bodies and how it affects us.

Alcohol does have a caloric content, but the amount of calories depends on the type of alcohol you are drinking and how much of it you drink. There are plenty of online calculators that can help you to see how many calories there are in the type of alcohol you are having. Don't forget to add the carbohydrates in from the pop or other beverages if you are having mixed drinks.

Your body uses a lot of water to digest alcohol and therefore can cause you to become dehydrated. If you remember, we learned earlier that muscles are made up of a lot of water. So having our bodies become dehydrated is detrimental to our muscle health and will not help us in the gym. If you are going to be drinking alcohol, be sure to drink water throughout the night to stay hydrated.

Other ways that alcohol can implicate your muscle building progress include: decreased strength, sleep deprivation, and impaired balance and motor skills. It also impacts muscle repair because protein metabolism is hindered when alcohol is in your system. As you can see by this list alcohol can affect our performance in the gym and hinder our body's ability to repair muscle and metabolize protein. The more alcohol you drink, the more all of these areas will be affected. Don't get me wrong, I love to have a beer or two after a long, hard day at work, but keep your goals in mind when you are consuming alcohol and don't let it get out of hand.

Alcohol is a depressant and in excess amounts can therefore cause you to become depressed and un-motivated. Speaking from personal experience, when I go out and drink, I normally feel down on myself and un-motivated for the next few days. Alcohol can affect people differently, but this is just how it affects me. This in turn has caused me to miss workouts in the gym and stray from my meal plan because I just don't have the motivation to do them and keep up with them. You don't need to get drunk to go out and have a good time. Keep it in moderation, remember the bigger plan, and stick to your goals.

Part 2 Supplements and More

Protein

Protein is the building block for all of the beefcakes out there. Without getting too technical, your body uses protein to repair your muscles after a workout. If you recall what working out does to your body, (creates small tears in your muscles) you should be able to put two and two together to realize that protein is what helps us to repair those muscle tears and create bigger and stronger muscles. Whatever doesn't kill you makes you stronger, right?

So how much protein should you eat in a day? Well that's a good question there Brian (I'm just hoping someone who is reading this book is named Brian because that would be sweet). The answer lies with your body weight. Generally, for a person who is doing weight training you are going to want to eat between 1 and 1.4 grams of protein per pound of body weight. If you weigh 170lbs you are going to want to eat between 170 grams and 238 grams of protein per day.

Easy right? Well maybe for experienced macro-counters, but what foods have protein? Here's a list of healthy foods that contain a good amount of protein in them;

- Chicken   - Tuna   - Greek Yogurt

- Navy Beans - Turkey   - Tilapia
- Steak   - Dried Lentils - Lean Ground Beef
- Egg Whites   - Halibut   - Quinoa

This is a good start, which will give you some variety, but there is a whole lot more out there than this, so be adventurous! Another option is to utilize protein shakes. You can purchase various size containers of protein powder at supplement stores and you can sometimes find them at your local grocery store or drug store. These shakes are very handy in helping you reach your daily protein needs, but I would recommend getting as much of your daily protein as possible from natural sources, like tuna or chicken. Look for whey protein products when you are buying protein powder. This type of protein has been proven to be most effective for recovery. I would not recommend protein bars. Although they are handy and on-the-go, a lot of them are expensive and the price doesn't justify the benefit. If you are going to utilize protein bars pay attention to the fat and carbohydrate content of the bar to make sure you know what you are putting into your body. Some of these bars can have a large amount of fat or carbs (sugar) to make them taste better.

Pre-Workout
Pretty self-explanatory, right? Not! A pre-workout is an energy booster you take before you workout to help you lift heavier weights and lift with more intensity. The

main ingredients in pre-workouts are usually a mixture of caffeine (which boosts energy), beta-alanine (which delays muscle fatigue), and L-arginine (which increases blood flow). It's not as simple as just taking it before every workout because your body will build up a tolerance to the powder and it will work slightly less effectively each time you take it. This causes the need to cycle your pre-workout. My recommendation is that you take your pre-workout before every workout for 2 months straight and then stop taking it for a week. After the week of working out without the pre-workout you can start up again and this should negate any tolerance build up that your body will experience. You can buy pre-workout powders from your local supplement store.

Multi-Vitamins

From now onwards a vitamin supplement should be an important part of your daily routine. Vitamins help our body to function correctly and keep us healthy. They can help us to fight off infections and colds as well which is very important because you don't want to be missing gym sessions because you're wrist deep in your own mucus. When looking to purchase a multi-vitamin look for something that has a good mixture of different vitamins. Definitely vitamins A., B., C., and D., as well as zinc. Also be sure to follow the instructions on the bottle. You may be surprised that those "One a Day" vitamins actually require you to take two pills a day.

Don't be ashamed to go for the gummy vitamins either. Buying them will not make you any less of an adult and they are delicious.

Fish Oil Pills

Fish oil pills are fantastic! These are an omega-3 fatty acid supplement that will help you immensely in your weight lifting journey. Fish oil pills help with muscle inflammation and studies suggest that they can also improve cognitive brain function. Keeping your muscles healthy and keeping your brain sharp, is there anything these pills can't do? Be sure to follow the recommended dosage and storage recommendations on the bottle.

Creatine

Creatine is found in red meats, such as beef, but is mostly depleted in the cooking process of the food. Creatine, as a supplement, can be purchased in powder form at supplement stores. Creatine sits in your muscles and pulls water in with it. After taking creatine you will have a store of water in your muscles which will help to keep you better hydrated and able to workout longer. This is a benefit because it will allow you to lift more weight for more repetitions due to your muscle's increased hydration. There has been no proven negative effects to taking creatine and it's considered to be a safe supplement in the fitness industry.

Creatine is easy to use, just take 5 grams daily with juice, a snack which has some simple sugars, or your protein powder and ignore any loading phases recommended on the tub. The human body, both male and female, can only absorb so much creatine in a serving. The 5 grams you take is enough that your body can absorb it all and not waste any. The loading phases on the tub are the manufacturer's way of getting you to use more of their product. If you take creatine in excess, which the loading phase suggests, it's not going to be beneficial to you and the excess creatine you take will just go to waste. You don't need to cycle this product because your body doesn't build up a tolerance to it, as with pre-workouts. I would not recommend taking this supplement until you have consistency in both your diet and workout routine. Having consistency in both of these areas will allow you to receive the biggest benefit from taking creatine. It's different for each individual as to when they become consistent and comfortable in their diet and workout routine. It's hard to put an exact number of months on when you should start taking creatine. Just be sure your diet and workout routine are in order and consistent before you start this supplement.

In my personal opinion all other supplements can be completely ignored for beginners. Other supplements will not provide you with enough bang for your buck and should only be utilized by people who have been working out for a very long time and need the extra help to push further or professionals who need all the help they can get to be at the top.

A Word On Steroids

It is almost human nature to try to do things the easy way and take shortcuts. Being efficient is different from taking shortcuts and this can be important in business as well as in the gym. Taking shortcuts and doing things the easy way can be unhealthy, especially in the gym. Steroids are a shortcut that a lot of people take who aren't willing to do all the work and put forth the effort, but want the results. Yes, indeed they still do have to put in a lot of work, but it's nothing compared to the hard work that someone who isn't on steroids has to put in. This means that there is also less of a reward as well. Would you rather do something knowing you did it the safe way and achieved your goals all on your own? Or would you rather put your health at risk just to get something done quicker? In the end you can build a lot more muscle mass when you are on steroids as opposed to doing it naturally, but the cost you have to pay is not worth it.

Steroids may help you to look good on the outside, but your body will actually be "rotting" on the inside. Without getting into any of the medical terms or specifics, studies are showing that the use of steroids can be detrimental to one's health and are unsafe. There is a reason that they are an illegal substance (in Canada anyways) and it's because the long term effects of steroid use are still relatively unknown. Yet, we still see countless amounts of users having bodily malfunctions at early ages and shortened lifespans of many elite body builders. Granted, there are always exceptions where people who have taken steroids for an extended period of time go on to live long and happy lives, but let's be serious, are we really ready to gamble with our lives?

Sure, steroids can do great things for people with various different health issues, but when used irresponsibly just to build muscle they can become dangerous. Having seen many people in my life hop on "gear" I can tell you that it's not healthy. So my strong recommendation to you is to do things the natural way and stay away from steroids. Trust me, when your hard work starts to pay off and you know that you did it all on your own, the sense of accomplishment will be far greater than what someone on steroids would feel. So choose to live a healthy life and stay away from steroids because in the end the short-term payoff isn't worth the long-term complications.

I would also strongly recommend watching documentaries online about steroid usage and the long term effects. There are many free videos online that you can search and they are all very informative.

How To Buy Protein

Step one: Go to the supplement store and buy a tub of protein… Oh if only it were that simple. Well, it still is simple, but there are a few key things that you should look for before you get out the credit card. The main keys you need to know are the two C's and the Q of protein: cost, contents, and quality.

Cost

Protein varies widely in the size of the tubs you can purchase and the cost of each tub. It will almost always make sense to go for the biggest tub you can find (with the exception of sale items) as this will give you the best deal. Companies want to sell you as much of their product as possible and they are willing to give you a little bit of a price break if you buy more of their product because it helps them to cut down on packaging costs etc. So whenever you are buying, make sure to buy the larger tub as it will save you money in the long run.

There is more to it than this though. The best way to find a cost effective protein is to do a cost per gram analysis when you are buying. This can be a little awkward to do if you are buying from a store, but it will save you money and get you the best bang for your buck. What you need to do is take the amount of servings in the tub (it will say on the tub) and multiply this by the number of grams of protein per serving. This will give you the amount of grams of protein in the tub. Now you simply need to divide the sale price by the total amount of grams of protein in the tub which will give you a cost per gram of protein. Doing this method will eliminate any differences in serving sizes or amount of servings per tub between brands.

For example,

Option 1: Let's say a tub of protein has 58 servings with 22 grams of protein per serving and is listed at $54.99. The cost per gram of protein can be calculated as follows:

58 servings * 22 grams of protein = 1276 grams of protein per tub

$54.99 / 1276 grams of protein per tub = $0.04 per gram rounded

This can easily be compared with any other brand or size of serving such as a smaller tub with more/less protein per serving and more/less servings per container:

Option 2: A tub of protein has 60 servings with 20 grams of protein per serving and is listed at $54.99.

60 servings * 20 grams of protein = 1200 grams of protein per tub

$54.99 / 1200 grams of protein per tub = $0.05 per gram rounded

As you can see from this comparison your best bet would be Option 1 as it has the lowest cost per gram for protein. Even though Option 2 has more servings, your best bet would be Option 1.

Contents

Let's be honest, there are some less than ideal products out there. But how do we decipher the good from the bad? To start off, I would recommend using whey protein as it is the best for promoting muscle recovery. Next we need to look at the fat and carbohydrate content in our protein. Anything more than 5 grams of fat per serving in your protein powder is a lot. Even 5 grams is quite a bit, but at 5 grams of fat per serving your protein is going to taste a lot better than if it had less. You also don't want too many carbohydrates in a serving either. For carbohydrates I would recommend having no more than 10 grams of carbs per serving as an absolute maximum, but the less you can get the better. The sugar in your protein will also make it taste better, but some products can go way overboard and have much of your serving be carbohydrates. Look for something with approximately a 2:1 protein to fats and carbs ratio. For example, if a tub of protein has 4 grams of fat and 8 grams of carbs it should have around 24 grams of protein per serving which would be a 2:1 ratio.

Quality

Any of the bigger name brands are usually a solid bet. Most of the products sold in supplement stores will be at least average quality, but always be sure to look for the best. I would worry about or question the quality of some items bought online, in grocery stores, in pharmacies, or products that have been significantly marked down. All of the good products are sold online, but there are also some really bad ones that don't make it into the stores and are sold exclusively online. With some of the supplements, especially ones being produced in third world countries, there is no guarantee that you are not going to be ingesting ground up rat protein. All joking aside stick to protein that is from a reputable source that you can trust for quality. The majority of protein comes from fish and there is no guarantee where the fish come from, but the protein that is developed by American or Canadian companies should at least have a standard of safety in place to ensure that their products are 100% safe to take. The tubs of protein sold in grocery stores and pharmacies often come in smaller quantities and have a lower amount of protein. First I would recommend buying at your local supplement store to support local business owners and secondly buying online from a reputable source if you are looking to save a little more money and have a greater variety. If you do buy online be sure to do your research because there is a chance that you may unknowingly purchase a sub-par product. Stick to big box supplement companies if you are buying online. Stay away from overpriced protein in the grocery store or pharmacy which may leave you disappointed.

Part 3 Time to Hit the Gym

Safety In The Gym – Know Your Body

There are many different ways in which safety becomes a factor in the gym. Between looking out for yourself and others around you, the importance of being aware and careful is second to no other. Listed below are a few safety concerns that you need to be aware of when you are in the gym:

- Use equipment properly and follow the instructions on the machines if you are using them. Improper use of the machinery can lead to the machine being damaged, or even worse, the injury of you or those around you. Machines can tip over when improperly used and it's important to use the properly.
- Don't throw the weights around in the gym. I have seen it so many times where someone has thrown or dropped the set of dumbbells or the barbell after the set and it has rolled and hit someone in the ankle. In the gym you not only have to worry about yourself, you also of to be conscious of the safety of others around you.
- Be aware of how you are feeling when you are working out. If something doesn't feel right to you it important to take a step back and make sure you are feeling good enough to lift. This can range anywhere from dizziness, a small pain in your back or leg, to

chest pain. If you really aren't feeling well, make sure to take the precautions to get yourself checked out.

- If you see someone who is doing something that is unsafe, be sure to let them know that what they are doing is unsafe or report to gym management before someone gets hurt. They might not like that you are telling them what to do, but just remember you are trying to help them and could be preventing them from injuring themselves or others.
- If you are unsure about anything in the gym be sure to ask either the trainers or other staff. Part of their job is to make sure everyone is safe and using the equipment properly and using proper form. If you don't know something, don't be afraid to ask for help.

The Timing of Your Workout

Many beginners ask, "What time of the day is the best to workout?" My answer is always the same, "It depends." You need to pick a time of day that can work into your schedule. Think of the time of day they you feel most motivated and ask yourself if that works with your schedule. You need to be able to work around your job and social obligations to find time to get into the gym. If you are a procrastinator it may be best to go first thing in the morning. There has been many times where I have told myself that I would go to the gym later in the day, but end up putting it off until it's too late. You need to take a look at your schedule and yourself and decide what time of the day works best for you.

There is no "perfect time" in the day to go to the gym. It is more important that you actually go to the gym than what time you go at. Personally, I find that when I go in the morning I am more productive throughout the day. I find that if I wait to go later in the day I don't have as much energy and drive when completing my workout. Obviously everyone is going to be different and what works for some, may not work for others. The important thing is that you find out what works for you and that you stick to your plan.

Equipment

Before you go and try to throw weights around like a beast, it's important to know what things are. Below are photos of different types of gym equipment that you are going to be using:

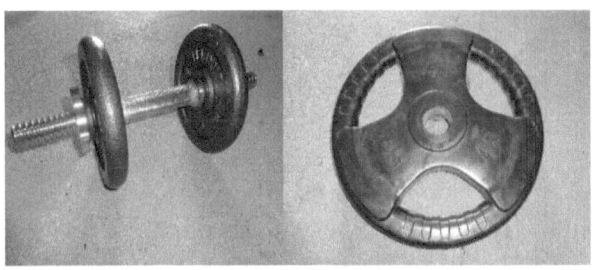

Dumbbell   Weight Plate

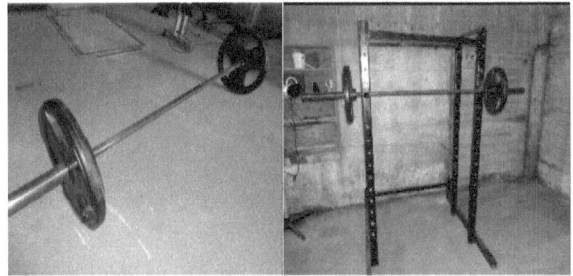

Barbell   Squat Rack

Repetitions and Sets

This is an easy concept that is awkwardly difficult to explain. One repetition (rep) is one movement in a set. For example one push up is one rep or one squat is one rep. A set is made up of multiple reps. An example would be if I did eight push ups in a row and then took a break, that would be one set. I could then move on to a second set of push ups, after that a third set and so on.

Size vs. Strength

Another decision you will have to make is whether you want to focus on building larger muscles while gaining a little bit of strength or gaining a lot of strength and a little bit of size. This will allow you to figure out which rep range you should work in.

Building Size

If you want to focus on building size I would recommend 8-12 reps per set. I would recommend around 15-20 sets per muscle group (Muscle groups may include: Lower body/abs, back/biceps, chest/shoulders/triceps). When you are doing this type of training you don't want to exhaust your muscles every single set. Do not perform so many reps that you can't do anymore. When you are completing a set you want to stay 1 rep away from failure throughout your workout. Pick a weight that you can do 10 reps with for the first set. Keep doing this weight until you can only get to 8 reps and would be unable to do a ninth and lower the weight a bit to keep your reps between 8-12 through your sets.

An example for clarification: Let's say you are doing 4 sets total of bicep curls.

> Set 1: You get to 10 reps with 20lbs dumbbells and you wouldn't be able to do an 11th rep.

> Set 2: You get to 10 reps again with the 20lbs dumbbells and wouldn't be able to do an 11th rep.

Set 3: Your biceps are beginning to get fatigued and you only make it to 8 reps and wouldn't be able to do a 9th rep.

Set 4: It's time to drop the weight a little bit so that you can stick to the 8-12 rep range because in all likelihood, your biceps will now be too fatigued to make it to 8 reps. So you need to drop down to the 15lbs dumbbells and try to get between 8-12 reps with them.

As you can see, even though you had to drop the weight by 5lbs for the last set, you still stuck to the 8-12 rep range. Over time you will gain strength as well and be able to progress towards 12 reps in your first set. At this point it's time to increase the weight of the dumbbell you are using to 25lbs and then drop the weight accordingly as you get to the point where you can do 8 reps, but not a 9th.

Generally, for dumbbells, they increase in increments of 5lbs so every time you move up the weight of your dumbbells it will be by 5lbs. For barbells there are speciality plates you can buy that will allow you to increase the amount of weight on the bar by 1 or 2lbs. Most gyms do not have these plates and you would have to purchase them yourself. As a beginner, I wouldn't recommend buying these plates as gains will come easy. These small weight plates are more for experienced weight lifters who are trying to squeeze every last drop out of their potential.

While you are building size, you are also gaining strength. The only catch is that because you are focused on gaining size, you will be gaining less strength than a person whose routine is focused solely on gaining strength.

Gaining Strength

If you want to focus on gaining strength I would recommend 3-6 reps per set. Start off with a weight that you can only do 5 reps with and work your way through the sets just like in the building size paragraph above. The only difference is that you are sticking to a rep range of 3-6 reps per set instead of 8-12 reps per set.

While you are gaining strength, you are also building some size. Again, the only catch is that you will not be building as much size as someone whose training is focused on building size.

Hybrid Training

Another option is to combine the two different training routines to try and obtain the best of both worlds. This consists of mixing up your routine with both strength training and size building exercises. For example you might do 2 sets of lighter weights in the 8-12 rep range and then another 2 sets with heavier weights in the 3-6 rep range.

Another option is to do strength training in the 3-6 rep range one week and size building training in the 8-12 rep range the next week. The options and combinations are endless and you are the one who gets to decide what you want to focus on. Just remember to track your workouts and continually progress to lifting heavier weights.

Isolation Movements and Compound Movements
An isolation movement puts greatest focus on a single muscle. For example, a bicep curl puts the greatest focus on your bicep muscles, even though you are still using other muscles including your forearms, back, shoulders, and core. Isolation movements are typically lighter weight movements because you are focusing on using one muscle to lift all of the weight.

A compound movement engages multiple muscles simultaneously to complete a rep. An example would be the bench press which would utilize the pectoral muscles (chest), shoulders, core, and triceps. Compound movements are much more taxing on your body and take a lot of energy to complete as you are using so many muscles at the same time. You typically use more weight in compound movements because you are using different muscles together which allows you to lift more weight.

Rest Periods

A rest period is the time you take between sets to let your muscles recover so you can perform the next set. These are important because; if you have too short of a rest period you will exhaust your muscles too quickly and won't get an effective workout and if you have too long of a rest period your muscles may become cold and you risk the chance of getting injured. So don't be hammering out sets like a jack rabbit or taking a 30 minute cell phone break between sets.

So what's the right amount of time for a rest period you ask? Well, I can answer that question easily: "It depends". This depends on the type of movement you are doing. If you are doing a compound movement which works out multiple muscles at once, like bench press, deadlifts, or squats, I would recommend taking a 2 minute rest period between sets. If you are doing an isolation type movement, like bicep curls, I would recommend only a 1.5 minute rest period between sets.

Taking rests between sets is very important and can often differentiate a good workout from a great one.

Using Momentum and Controlling the Weights

As a weightlifter, it would appear that momentum is your friend because it allows you to lift more weight, right? Wrong! Momentum is your enemy and it will kill your gains. Momentum is the swinging of weights and utilization of other muscles to help you lift weights that you wouldn't normally be able to lift through proper form. By taking my advice and not using momentum you are going to become much bigger and stronger.

Check your ego at the door ladies and gentlemen, it doesn't matter if you're using 10lbs for dumbbell curls, as long as you are controlling the weights, utilizing the muscles that the exercise is meant to target, and sticking to your rep range you are on the right path. Controlling the weights throughout the exercise is key to getting the full benefit from the lift. Go at a steady pace that is not too fast and not too slow. Personally, I like to spend roughly 2-3 seconds lifting the weight up and 2-3 seconds setting the weight back down. This allows me to control the weights I'm lifting and to target the muscles that I should be using for the lift.

This leads me to my next rant. Don't look at what other people are doing in the gym. It doesn't matter if Big Tony in the corner over there has 400lbs on the bench. You are not Tony and you shouldn't be comparing yourself to him because you are both at different places in your journey. It's a slow process and the only person you should be worried about is yourself. Although a healthy rivalry can help you push yourself in the gym, don't compete against others. Just focus on bettering yourself and doing the best you can. Increase the amount of weight you lifted or the number of reps you did in your last workout rather than comparing yourself to others in the gym. Compare yourself to yourself and try to improve and be better every time you hit the gym.

Range of Motion

The range of motion is the range in which the weights are supposed to travel through your lift from the start of the lift to the finish. During every rep you want to utilize the full range of motion for that exercise. For example; if you are doing deadlifts the range of motion would be from when the weights are on the ground, to the point where you are fully locked out (or vertical), and back down to where the weights are on the ground.

Not doing the full range of motion would be picking the bar up off the ground lifting it halfway up and putting it back down. This is a bad habit to get into because for one, you aren't fully utilizing your muscles throughout the lift and two, it can be dangerous to stop part way through a rep because you can injure yourself.

Similarly, you do not want to over extend your muscles and go out of the range of motion either. When you are doing a deadlift you do not want to over extend your back and be leaning backwards at the top of the lift. Over extending your muscles will lead to injury, which we want to avoid.

Sticking within the range of motion is key for properly utilizing your muscles and for avoiding injuries.

Weight Training For Dumbbells

Cheat Reps: What They Are and Why You Shouldn't Do Them

A "cheat rep" is a term used for an improperly executed rep by means of using momentum or by not completing the full range of motion. Basically, you are either getting the weight up by any means possible or not doing the full range of motion. You are going to want to stay away from cheat reps for one simple reason; they are impossible to track. Sure, it feels like you are absolutely ripped after getting that one last cheat rep in and you have the feeling that you really pushed it by totally exhausting your muscles. But, what are you going to write on your spreadsheet when tracking your workout? "I did bicep curls, did 73.6% of the range of motion, swung my arm like a pendulum at a 35 degree angle, and I engaged my triceps muscles throughout 13% of the lift". No. It doesn't work like this. You can't accurately track this rep to follow it up in future workouts. "Progressive overload" is tracking exactly what you have done and improving in the next workout with more reps or more weight. When you do cheat reps you are hindering your progression because you can't properly track them.

Yes, it's true. It does happen to all of us. Sometimes we accidentally over extend ourselves and are unable to complete a full rep or have to engage other muscles to complete the rep, but this issue has an easy fix. If you don't properly execute a rep at the end of your set, don't record it as a full rep. Try to get that extra rep next week and make sure you are doing it properly. This will help you to keep your tracking accurate and your progression smooth.

Proper Breathing Techniques

Whoever thought that breathing could be so important? Breathing is something that we do naturally without even thinking about it, but in the gym it serves an important purpose: getting enough oxygen to your muscles. To get the most out of each and every set you are going to want to make sure your breath-taking abilities are on point. Specifically, I mean inhaling during the eccentric portion of the lift and exhaling during the concentric portion of the lift. The eccentric portion of the lift means when your muscles are lengthening (when you are lowering down the bar to your chest during bench press) and concentric portion of the lift means when your muscles are shortening (when you are pushing the bar up from your chest during bench press). For example, if you are doing bench press, the eccentric portion of the lift is going to be the part where you lower the bar to your chest. At this point you are going to want to be breathing in air as you lower the bar down. Once the bar is to your chest you are going to want to begin to exhale and push at the same time to complete the concentric portion of the lift. Exhaling during the concentric portion of your lift will help you be more explosive and allow you to lift more weight as well.

The breathing techniques for a squat are slightly different. Once you get yourself set on your shoulders you are going to want to take in a breath and squat down to the lowest position without breathing out. You will want to have air in your belly so you can push it out throughout the downward portion of the lift. When you push back up you can begin to breathe out until you reach the position that you started in. The key is to not take any air in or let any air out while you are squatting the weight down. You need to keep your abs tight with air in your belly pressing outward. Once you get to the low point of the lift and start to stand back up you can begin to exhale.

A helpful to check if you are bringing air into your belly instead of your chest is to breathe in and if your shoulders rise it means that you are bringing air into your chest. If your shoulders stay at the same level, it means that you are bringing air into your belly.

A weightlifting belt (described below) can be a handy tool while doing squats because you can push your belly out against the belt for increased stabilization.

Focusing On the Muscles You Are Training
This is a simple but important tip that will help you to workout effectively. Making sure that you are using the

correct muscles during a lift is often overlooked during the workout. This will allow you to target the exact muscle that you are supposed to be training to get the most effective workout for that particular muscle. An example of this happening is when you are doing lateral raises for your shoulders, we can sometimes subconsciously engage our bicep and triceps muscles to help us with the lift. Now, granted, there is always going to be a little help from your bicep and triceps muscles during this exercise because our body's muscles always work together to complete tasks. It is important, however, to make sure that your shoulders are doing most of the work and that your biceps and triceps aren't taking over the movement. Be conscious of the muscles you are using when you are doing a lift and keep in mind proper form because this will help to limit having other muscles in your body take over the lift. This can be key in maintaining muscle balance as well which will be discussed next.

Muscle Imbalances – What Are They and How Can They be fixed?

A muscle imbalance occurs when a muscle on one side of your body is bigger than on the other side of your body. For example, someone's left bicep may be noticeably bigger than their right bicep. There are several causes for this including a person doing more reps or using more weight on one side than the other or by using improper form on one side of the body as opposed to the other. As with compound movements, like the bench press with a barbell, one side of your body could be pushing more of the weight than the other side even though you perceive the bar as going up level.

If you think you have a muscle imbalance, don't only judge by what you see in the mirror as sometimes the lighting in the room and our minds can trick us. Grab a tape measure so that you can get accurate results and record what you find so that you can track your progress over time. There are a few different ways that muscle imbalances can occur, but how do we fix them?

The most important thing, like with anything in bodybuilding, is to be patient. Don't look for a quick fix because you may get injured or make things worse. I'm going to first recommend what not to do; DO NOT use less weight on one side or do more reps on one side in an attempt to grow one muscle faster. This can cause muscle strains and can be very dangerous for the lifter as it makes the weight very difficult to balance. Here's what you should do: check your form using a mirror or video camera, ensure that you are using the same amount of weight on both sides, focus on controlling the weight, and be conscious that you are using the muscles you are supposed to be using. In the case of one of your pectoral muscles being larger than the other, I would recommend switching from a barbell to using dumbbells for your lifts to ensure that each side of your body is lifting the same amount while you are pressing.

It will take some time to correct muscle imbalances, but if you stick to proper form and are conscious of the muscles you are using when lifting, it should be easy to overcome. Be patient, Michael Angelo's "David" was not perfectly sculpted in a day and neither will your body.

Mind Over Matter

Believing is achieving. Have you ever heard experts say that? Well, the reason they say that is because it's true. Truly believing you can do something and having confidence in yourself will help you achieve things that you never thought you could. This applies to your workouts in the gym as well. It is tough when you are first starting out to have confidence in yourself because you are in a new place which is uncomfortable. You need to work on building yourself up over time and celebrate both the big triumphs and little triumphs you have in the gym. When you have confidence in yourself and believe you can do something, you are much more likely to achieve your goal. Be positive going into every lift and you will be surprised at what you can achieve. You might be asking yourself "How is mind over matter and confidence going to help me in the gym?" Well here's how:

Let's compare two people, Larry and Joe. They are both going to try to push 135lbs on the bench press. Both Larry and Joe are equally strong and experienced in the gym. Larry is not confident in his abilities and doesn't think he will be able to complete the lift. Joe on the other hand believes in his abilities and is sure he can successfully lift the weight. Who do you think will be successful in lifting the weight? That's right, Joe will be successful because he isn't going in with a mindset that he can't lift the weight. With that being said, I don't want you, as a beginner, going into the gym and throwing 400lbs on the bar believing you can lift it. Don't get me wrong, I'm glad you are taking my advice to heart, but you are going to hurt yourself. Start off within your means, work your way up, and track everything you lift!

Here is an example from when I was beginning my weightlifting journey. I was doing the bench press and I was going for a 1 rep max personal record. I had two 35lb weights, and two 25lb weights on the bar for a total of 120lbs on the bar. That seemed like a lot of weight to me because they were bigger plates and I was unsure of myself. I ended up failing the lift and had to get help lifting the bar back up. The next set I said to myself, "OK, well I'll put the 45lb weights on the bar and just add a couple smaller weights because I know I can do that". So I put on two 45lb weights, two 10lb weights, and two 5lb weights for a total of 120lbs. That's right the exact same amount! Sometimes I don't math so good. Guess what happened? I completed the lift with ease and didn't realize until after that it was actually the same amount of weight that I had on the bar when I failed. My perception of how much bigger the weights looked on the first lift affected my performance because I didn't believe I could do it. My perception of how the smaller weights made the bar look like it was not as heavy affected my performance because I believed that I could do the lift. This is a true story that happened to me, I wouldn't feed you some fake motivational information. It is true and a great testimony to how having confidence in yourself and using mind over matter can help you in the gym.

Let's Talk About Consistency

Consistency is key in the world of weight lifting. To not do the time is the crime in this case. Being consistent means bringing the same or higher level of intensity to your workout every day, as well as working out on a consistent basis. If you think you are going to walk into the gym once a week for an hour and get the results that you want, you are sadly mistaken. Keep yourself motivated to workout and put in the time. This is not a process that takes a workout here and there. No, it takes months and years of consistently hitting the weights at least three times a week. So pull up your boots and let's do some work!

The key factor is to consistently bring the same amount of intensity to your workouts. If you are just going to phone it in one week and do half of your normal amount of reps with less weight, you might as well stay home because you are just spinning your tires. Stay motivated to bring the same amount of intensity every week and you will see results.

Drop Sets and Pyramid Sets

Drop sets are an exercise where you slowly move towards muscle exhaustion by completing reps with a specific amount of weight until you start to feel fatigued. At this point you lower the amount of weight you are lifting to complete more reps and repeat. An example of a drop set for biceps would be:

Bicep Curl Set 1 – 10 reps 30lbs

Bicep Curl Set 2 – 10 reps 20lbs

Bicep Curl Set 3 – 10 reps 15lbs

Bicep Curl Set 4 – 10 reps 10lbs

You need to complete each set directly after the previous set without a break for this to be successful. Obviously the amount of reps you get with each weight is going to vary slightly. This example gives you an idea of how a drop set works. Doing drop sets allows you to recruit different muscle fibres in the muscle you are working out by exhausting some muscle fibres in that muscle and using new ones when you lower the weights. You can do as many sets as you feel comfortable doing, but do pay attention to what your body is telling you so that you don't get injured. Drop sets can be a fun change from your regular workout and can help you to build muscle, but they aren't necessary in your regular workout.

A pyramid set is the reverse of the drop set. In a pyramid set you start off with lighter weight and move up in weight with each set. With every set you are able to do less reps with each increase in weight. A pyramid set would resemble this:

Bicep Curl Set 1 – 15 reps 10lbs

Bicep Curl Set 2 – 12 reps 15lbs

Bicep Curl Set 3 – 8 reps 20lbs

Bicep Curl Set 4 – 5 reps 30lbs

Bicep Curl Set 5 – 1 rep 40lbs

Again, the amount of reps and weight you are able to use will vary. The end goal of the pyramid set is to exhaust your muscle to the point where you can only get one rep with the weight you are using. You can work pyramid sets into your workouts, but they aren't necessary by any means.

I would recommend doing drop sets or pyramid sets at the end of your workout and I would only recommend them for isolation exercises. You don't want to totally exhaust your muscles at the beginning or middle of your workout. It can be risky doing compound movements for drop/pyramid sets when you are totally exhausted as there are a lot of moving parts and you are lifting a large amount of weight. Don't over-use these training methods because they do take a toll on your body. Your body needs to be able to recover and when you do these types of workout constantly, it can be hard for your body to keep up and repair itself.

Part 4 Getting Ready for your Workout

Warming Up – Why It Is Important

Warming up is like studying for a math test. The more effectively you study, the better you are going to do on the test. If you don't study at all the more likely you are to fail. Just like the more effectively you warm up, the better your workout will be and the less chance there will be for you to fail (get injured). It is crucial to put in the time to get warmed up before you start slinging weights around.

There are a couple different things you should do to get warmed up for your workout. Start off with some light stretching. Stick to dynamic stretching before your workout. I go through this below. The next step is to do a couple sets with light weights to get your body ready for the motions that you will be completing. For example, if you are going to be doing bench press, start off by pressing just the bar and then do a set with 10lbs on each side of the bar before moving to your regular weight.

The purpose of warming up is to get your body ready for your workout and to lessen your chances of getting injured. So study for that test and get ready for the success that comes with proper preparation!

When To Do Cardio

Cardiovascular work, like running or skating, is great for your body, but it can inhibit your muscle gains a couple different ways. The first is that it burns calories that could be used for muscle gains. If you burn 200 calories doing a cardio workout and this puts you into a caloric deficit, then you will not be building as much muscle as you possibly can. To remedy this, you can consume 200 extra calories in food to make-up for the calories that you burnt while exercising. The second is that it uses up valuable energy that you will need for your weight lifting. When you do intense cardio before a weightlifting session, you are using up energy that you need to lift the weights and complete your workout effectively. If you are going to do cardio, do it after your workout and stick to only doing it a few times a week. Warming up is always a good idea, but if you are going to use it to get warmed up, stick to something light and do no more than 5 minutes.

Stretching – Is It Really Important?

The answer to the question in the above title is "YES it is important!" Stretching will allow you to increase your range of motion with some exercises and help you to avoid injury by warming you up and increasing muscle dexterity so that your muscles can handle more stress in different positions. Stretching will not cause you to lose muscle. It will help you increase performance in the gym and help you to stay healthy so that you don't miss any workouts and/or impede your progress.

There are two types of stretching: Static Stretches and Dynamic Stretches.

Static Stretches

Static stretching is when you gradually increase the length of your muscle to an elongated position and hold it for 30 seconds. 30 seconds will give your muscles enough of a stretch without putting undue stress on the muscle you are stretching. An example would be, from a standing position, grab your foot and pull it towards your butt to elongate the quadricep muscle in your leg and hold it at a point where you can feel your muscle stretch and hold this position for 30 seconds. Over time you will see and feel yourself become more flexible and the stretches will start to feel good instead of a little painful. It's normal to feel a little pain or discomfort when you first start your stretching journey, but be sure to not push it so far that you injure yourself. Static stretching is meant to be done when you are resting, so it's not a good idea to do this before a workout. I would recommend doing it in the morning when you wake up, or slightly after you have finished a workout. There are many videos online on how to do static stretches. Find one that works for you and make sure to pay attention to your form and completing the stretch correctly.

Dynamic Stretches

Dynamic stretching is the type of stretching that you need to do before working out to get yourself warmed up. Dynamic stretching is stretching with movement. It is when you use your muscles and momentum to move your muscles to the point where you would feel a stretch during your static stretching. We've all seen runners kicking their foot out in front of them to stretch out their hamstrings. What they are doing is kicking their leg up in the air so it fully extends to the point that it stretches out their hamstrings. Arm circles are also a form of dynamic stretching which can activate your shoulder, arm, and chest muscles. Dynamic stretching should be done before a workout because it will give your muscles a quick stretch, as well as get blood flowing to your muscles. This will help you to get properly warmed up for your workout and help you to avoid injury in the gym. There are lots of different types of dynamic stretches and you should focus more on doing stretches that directly relate to the workout you're doing. It is still important to do full body dynamic stretching before a workout, but it doesn't make sense to focus heavily on dynamic stretches for your hamstrings when you are doing a chest workout. For examples of dynamic stretches, check out one of the many videos online and remember to stick to the proper form noted in the videos.

One of the many mistakes that I made when I was starting out was not paying enough attention to stretches. I battled some annoying injuries, was rigid in the gym, and had a lot of set-backs due to me not working on my flexibility. Stretches can seem annoying to do, and they can be, but stick to them because they will pay off and help you on your journey. You wouldn't write an exam without studying, would you? Well maybe some of us would, but we wouldn't expect to get a very high grade. Do the stretches, aim for the high grade, and results will follow. Trust me!

Before Your Workout

Before your workout you want to ensure that you are not only physically prepared, but also mentally prepared as well. This means being in the right mind frame to train and being ready to put in the work. Getting properly warmed up for your workout is part of the battle, but there are also things like pre-workouts that we can to take before the workout that will help us as well.

A pre-workout isn't mandatory, but it can help you in the gym. I can't even count the amount of times I see people improperly using pre-workout mixtures in the gym. This is not something that you should be sipping on throughout your workout. Your pre-workout needs to be taken 15-30 minutes before you workout in order to metabolize the contents and give you the energy you need. When you drink it while you are working out you will not be getting the full effect of the pre-workout because your body hasn't had enough time to process and absorb the pre-workout. If you are going to take a pre-workout be sure to take it before your workout begins and not during. You should be drinking water during your workouts, not pre-workout.

Be sure to have everything that you will need during the workout handy while you are in the gym. Whether this be in a bag or kept at the gym, it is important to be prepared. The reason that this is important is because you don't want to be running to the change room or your car looking for gloves, straps, different shoes etc. while you are in the middle of your workout. While getting these things someone else could take the machine you were on causing you to have to wait or your muscles could even tighten back up if you take too long which could lead to injury. It's just not efficient to be spending extra time gathering things that you could easily just have brought with you in a bag.

Recovery After Working Out

The first step to recovery begins with your workout. Don't annihilate your body every single workout. You want to push your body to the point where you will stimulate muscle growth, but not to the point where you are extremely sore for days and have a tough time recovering. The effects of constantly pushing your body as hard as it can go may be detrimental to your body building goals. Some recovery advocates suggest that your body stops its focus on rebuilding your muscles bigger and starts to focus on just repairing the damage to your muscles caused by the workout. Although the feeling of pushing yourself as hard as you can go is amazing, it's important to realize that this might not be the most beneficial thing for your body.

Be sure to keep in mind what you are eating and make sure your body has what it needs to recover. Make sure you are getting enough protein and that your diet is on point. This well help you to recover faster.

On your off days, be sure to get your body in light motion. Whether this is just walking the dog or doing some light stretches, it is very helpful to recovery to get your body in motion and get your blood flowing.

Be sure you are getting enough sleep and try to lessen the amount of stress in your life. Both of these will help your body to recover faster and more effectively. Your body does the most of its recovery while you are asleep, so it's important to get enough sleep to allow your body the time to recover. Your stress level is the direct result of your surroundings. When you are mentally stressed and start to add physical stress from going to the gym to your life this can be a recipe for injury and/or poor workouts.

The Gear

There are plenty of different items you can bring to the gym. Here I will name a few useful items that you should think about picking up at your local sports store.

Chalk – Chalk can be really handy for helping you with your grip while doing exercises like deadlifts. It helps to keep the bar from slipping out of your hands. You rub it on your hands or other areas which come into contact with the bar. Not all gyms allow chalk because it can be messy, so check with the gym staff before using this product.

Lifting Straps – Not necessary for the beginner, but definitely helpful when you get into the heavier weights. These straps help you with your grip strength and allow you to lift more weight for more reps without you losing grip. Simply attach to your wrists and wrap around the bar to use the straps. You can also follow the instructions that come with the straps.

Lifting Belt – A weightlifting belt can help you to keep your back in the right position while you are lifting heavy weights. Belts help you with stabilization and can help you to reduce stress on your spine. Typically, belts are used during deadlifts and squats. To use the belt properly it has to be tight around your midsection, above your belt line. You don't want it to be so tight that you can't breathe, but you do want it to be tight enough that you can press your core muscles (abs) up against the belt to help stabilize yourself. Studies have shown that lifting belts can help improve form as well as help to increase the amount of weight you can lift. This is a solid investment when you get into lifting heavier weights.

Gloves – Some people opt to wear gloves in the gym. Gloves help to prevent you from developing calluses on your hands while in the gym. Some people see these calluses as a sense of pride and accomplishment while others see them as painful and annoying. Decide what type of person you are and purchase accordingly.

Shoes – There are shoes that are designed specifically for weightlifting. These typically have flat, wide soles and are fairly pricey. These are not necessary for the beginner. The shoes you wear in the gym should have flat soles which will help you complete movements like squats and deadlifts with better and safer form. It is important that these shoes don't have a thick heel which will pitch you forward. A lot of running shoes have this forward pitch. If you don't want to buy lifting shoes I would recommend skateboarding shoes as they almost all have flat soles, are not pitched forward, and can be fairly inexpensive. For cardio activities I would recommend not using your lifting shoes. Running shoes are your best bet as they are designed to keep you comfortable while running and promote proper running form.

Knee and Elbow Braces – Again these aren't really necessary for the beginning lifter, but can be helpful when you get to heavier weights. These braces help to stabilize your elbows and knees while lifting heavy weights.

Foam Roller – Foam rollers are used by many professional lifters. They are used to eliminate scar tissue in your muscles by applying force to affected areas and relieving tension. Foam rolling can be incredibly painful at first, but will start to feel good once you do it a few times. I have personally been astounded at the work that foam rollers can do. Muscle pain or discomfort that I have had for days or weeks can often be eliminated by one foam rolling session. If you buy one, make sure to get one with a plastic insert in the centre. This gives it a little rigidity and allows it to keep its form. The foam rollers which are all foam will lose their shape after time and be less effective.

A final word on equipment refers to the type of clothing you wear. You will want to wear something that is comfortable for you, but doesn't inhibit your workout. For example you shouldn't wear shorts so tight that you are uncomfortable and you shouldn't wear a t-shirt so baggy that it gets caught up in the cable machine. Find something in the middle that you are comfortable wearing and will be happy to wear.

Gym Etiquette

Before you start pumping the iron it's important to learn some basic rules that you should abide by while within the walls of the gym. Here are my top ten gym etiquette rules to help you avoid making enemies in the gym:

1. Don't curl in the squat rack. You know that big bar that lies across that metal contraption? Yes, that one. That area is solely meant for squats. If you want to do curls I urge you to just pick up a set of dumbbells or use the smaller barbells that your gym has provided for you.

2. Don't be a grunter. You would be surprised about the number of guttural, beastly noises that come from people's bodies when they are in the gym. Keep your grunting to a minimum. It annoys everyone and in the end it really just sounds like you are trying to have a bowel movement.

3. Wipe your machines down. Your gym will provide you with some sort of towel/spray combination or sanitary wipe. Wipe those sweat marks down after using a machine if you've left any. When machines aren't wiped down, harmful bacteria can form on them and they can start to smell.

4. Don't lollygag on the machines. Unless you have your own personal gym, make your time on each machine snappy. Don't take overly long on the

machine. Everyone has to use them so be courteous to the other gym-goers.

5. Don't be on your phone at the gym. Business calls and emails are best left to be done at the office. You're at the gym for one reason and it's not to catch-up on work.

6. Wear headphones. Did it ever occur to you that not everyone wants to listen to your Caribbean trip-hop music? Use headphones and keep everyone around you happy. There are awesome wireless headphones that work great for the gym!

7. Keep it to small talk. No one, I repeat NO ONE in the gym wants to hear your life story. Keep it to a short hello and leave the gossip for after the gym. This isn't social hour ladies and gentlemen.

8. Don't drop or slam the weights. You just did 10 reps of dumbbell press with the 80lb dumbbells? Well that's pretty impressive, but it doesn't give you the right to drop the weights or toss them to the sides. Not only is it dangerous for others around you for you to do this, it's also disrespectful to the gym owner and to the other gym-goers around you. Throwing and slamming the weights can damage them and they aren't cheap, not to mention the high chance of injuring others around you with weights tumbling across the floor.

9. Put the weights away when you are done. Nothing drives me crazier than when I walk into a gym and I see the weights are scattered all over the place. Clean up after yourself and put the weights you use back in their designated area.

10. Wash your gym clothes frequently. Nobody likes the smell of your sweaty gym shirt wafting into their face when you walk by. Wash your clothes weekly so you aren't causing people to faint in the gym.

Part 5 Workout Spreadsheets and Game Plan

Getting Started

So I bet you're ready to start swinging some dumbbells around and firing off some squats eh? Easy there, you're still a beginner. The first two weeks of your training career I want you to stick to using the machines in your gym. Let's face it, if you were trying skateboarding for the first time would you drop in from a twenty foot halfpipe? Or would you try balancing on the ground first? Be smart about it and don't get too over-eager. The machines are a safe way to start as they don't put you at as much risk for injury because you aren't trying to balance heavy weights throughout the movement. The machines are designed to focus on specific muscles which is a great way to start for beginners.

The First and Second Week

The first week you will start off by going to the gym three days. Go the first day, take a day off, go the third day, take a day off, and go the fifth day, and then take the next two days off. This will allow your body sufficient time to recover between workouts. In the first week you are going to do full body workouts and limited amounts of sets for each exercise.

I want you to focus on hitting your rep range. Start off light and move up until you find out how much you can lift. It may be difficult at first to figure out how much you can lift, but it will become easier as time goes on.

Remember to write down all the sets that you do and how many reps as well as the amount of weight. Here is a simple spreadsheet that you can follow for the first and second week:

Week 1 & 2 Workout				
	Week 1		Week 2	
Exercise	Weight	# of Reps	Weight	# of Reps
Example	100lbs	12 reps	110lbs	11 reps
Rowing Machine Set 1				
Rowing Machine Set 2				
Shoulder Press Machine Set 1				
Shoulder Press Machine Set 2				
Chest Press Machine Set 1				
Chest Press Machine Set 2				
Leg Curl Machine Set 1				
Leg Curl Machine Set 2				
Leg Extension Machine Set 1				
Leg Extension Machine Set 2				
Bicep Curl Machine Set 1				
Bicep Curl Machine Set 2				
Tricep Extension Machine Set 1				
Tricep Extension Machine Set 2				

This is a very good starting point. It is about as close to a full body workout as you can get without it being too much in the first week. It's important to start off slow so that your body can adjust to these new activities you are putting it through. Believe me, you will be very sore after the first week and it will take a couple of days for the pain to go away, but this is good pain and your body will get used to doing the workouts over time. When your body gets more into the swing of things you will be less sore after going to the gym, trust me.

The Third and Fourth Week

The third and fourth weeks get a little more complex. We are still going to stick to the machines, but we are going to move up to four gym sessions in a week and focus on a different muscle group in each workout. **Workout 1** will be **chest and triceps**. This is a push workout and we group your chest muscles in with your tricep muscles because they are both used in a lot of the movements you will be doing. **Workout 2** will be **back and biceps**. Again these two are grouped together because they are also used together in a lot of the movements you will be doing. **Workout 3** will be **legs and abs**. This is the perfect combination because when you do a lot of the leg exercises you will also be engaging your abdominal muscles as well. **Workout 4** is **shoulders**.

In the third week, try to better the amount of reps or weight you did in the previous week in the exercises that you will be repeating next week. The following are spreadsheets for the 8 workouts you will be doing in your third and fourth weeks of training.

Week 3 & 4 - Workout 1 – Chest and Triceps				
	Week 3		Week 4	
Exercise	Weight	# of Reps	Weight	# of Reps
Chest Press Machine Set 1				
Chest Press Machine Set 2				
Chest Press Machine Set 3				
Chest Fly Machine Set 1				
Chest Fly Machine Set 2				
Chest Fly Machine Set 3				
Push-ups Set 1				
Push-ups Set 2				
Push-ups Set 3				
Tricep Extension Machine Set 1				
Tricep Extension Machine Set 2				
Tricep Extension Machine Set 3				
Rope Tricep Extension Set 1				
Rope Tricep Extension Set 2				
Rope Tricep Extension Set 3				
End of Workout 1. Good Job! You go girl! I mean Guy!				

Week 3 & 4 - Workout 2 – Back and Biceps				
	Week 3		Week 4	
Exercise	Weight	# of Reps	Weight	# of Reps
Pull-ups Set 1				
Pull-ups Set 2				
Pull-ups Set 3				
Rowing Machine Set 1				
Rowing Machine Set 2				
Rowing Machine Set 3				
Lat Pull Down Machine Set 1				
Lat Pull Down Machine Set 2				
Lat Pull Down Machine Set 3				
Bicep Curl Machine Set 1				
Bicep Curl Machine Set 2				
Bicep Curl Machine Set 3				
Dumbbell Bicep Curl Set 1				
Dumbbell Bicep Curl Set 2				
Dumbbell Bicep Curl Set 3				
End of Workout 2. Keep up the good work stud!				

Week 3 & 4 - Workout 3 – Legs and Abs				
	Week 3		Week 4	
Exercise	Weight	# of Reps	Weight	#of Reps
Leg Press Machine Set 1				
Leg Press Machine Set 2				
Leg Press Machine Set 3				
Leg Curl Machine Set 1				
Leg Curl Machine Set 2				
Leg Curl Machine Set 3				
Leg Extension Machine Set 1				
Leg Extension Machine Set 2				
Leg Extension Machine Set 3				
Dumbbell Lunges Set 1				
Dumbbell Lunges Set 2				
Dumbbell Lunges Set 3				
Sit-ups Set 1				
Sit-ups Set 2				
Sit-ups Set 3				
Leg Raises Set 1				
Leg Raises Set 2				
Leg Raises Set 3				
End of Workout 3. Grab some protein and relax! You deserve it!				

Week 3 & 4 - Workout 4 – Shoulders				
	Week 3		Week 4	
Exercise	Weight	# of Reps	Weight	# of Reps
Shoulder Press Machine Set 1				
Shoulder Press Machine Set 2				
Shoulder Press Machine Set 3				
Neutral Grip Overhead Dumbbell Press Set 1				
Neutral Grip Overhead Dumbbell Press Set 2				
Neut. Grip Over. DB Press 3				
Dumbbell Lateral Raise Set 1				
Dumbbell Lateral Raise Set 2				
Dumbbell Lateral Raise Set 3				
Dumbbell Shrugs Set 1				
Dumbbell Shrugs Set 2				
Dumbbell Shrugs Set 3				
Cable Face Pulls Set 1				
Face Pulls Set 2				
Face Pulls Set 3				
End of Workout 4. It`s been a hell of a week hasn`t it?				

Weeks 5 and 6… and Beyond!

These are the weeks that we start to get into the more complex movements like the barbell bench press, the deadlift, the squat, and the barbell standing military press. These exercises are meant to target many muscles in the same movement and put more strain on your muscles which will help you to build muscle faster.

To start off, I will give you a table of the exercises I want you to do and then there will be a link to the new exercises which will show you how to complete the exercise with proper form. Don't worry, these guides are short and precise as well as easy to understand. So here we go, time for you to enter the big leagues!

Week 5 & 6 & Beyond - Workout 1 – Chest and Triceps				
	Week 5		Week 6	
Exercise	Weight	# of Reps	Weight	# of Reps
Barbell Bench Press Set 1				
Bench Press Set 2				
Bench Press Set 3				
Barbell Bench Press Set 4				
Incline Dumbbell Bench Press Set 1				
Incline Dumbbell Bench Press Set 2				
Incline Dumbbell Bench Press Set 3				
Chest Fly Machine Set 1				
Chest Fly Machine Set 2				
Chest Fly Machine Set 3				
Tricep Extension Machine Set 1				
Tricep Extension Machine Set 2				
Tricep Extension Machine Set 3				
Rope Tricep Extension Set 1				
Rope Tricep Extension Set 2				
Rope Tricep Extension Set 3				
Link to Barbell Bench Press Guide: https://www.youtube.com/watch?v=iDPHd02VaIg				

Week 5 & 6 & Beyond - Workout 2 – Back and Biceps				
	Week 5		Week 6	
Exercise	Weight	# of Reps	Weight	# of Reps
Deadlift Set 1				
Deadlift Set 2				
Deadlift Set 3				
Deadlift Set 4				
Pull-ups Set 1				
Pull-ups Set 2				
Pull-ups Set 3				
Rowing Machine Set 1				
Rowing Machine Set 2				
Rowing Machine Set 3				
Lat Pull Down Machine Set 1				
Lat Pull Down Machine Set 2				
Lat Pull Down Machine Set 3				
Dumbbell Bicep Curl Set 1				
Dumbbell Bicep Curl Set 2				
Dumbbell Bicep Curl Set 3				
Dumbbell Hammer Curl Set 1				
Dumbbell Hammer Curl Set 2				
Dumbbell Hammer Curl Set 3				
Link to Deadlifts guide: https://www.youtube.com/watch?v=sCt8bW1ngTQ				

Week 5 & 6 & Beyond - Workout 3 – Legs and Abs				
	Week 5		Week 6	
Exercise	Weight	# of Reps	Weight	# of Reps
Barbell Squats Set 1				
Barbell Squats Set 2				
Barbell Squats Set 3				
Barbell Squats Set 4				
Leg Curl Machine Set 1				
Leg Curl Machine Set 2				
Leg Curl Machine Set 3				
Leg Extension Machine Set 1				
Leg Extension Machine Set 2				
Leg Extension Machine Set 3				
Dumbbell Lunges Set 1				
Dumbbell Lunges Set 2				
Dumbbell Lunges Set 3				
Sit-ups Set 1				
Sit-ups Set 2				
Sit-ups Set 3				
Leg Raises Set 1				
Leg Raises Set 2				
Leg Raises Set 3				
Link to Barbell Squats Guide: https://www.youtube.com/watch?v=Ns8Dkq6c1os				

Week 5 & 6 & Beyond - Workout 4 – Shoulders				
	Week 5		Week 6	
Exercise	Weight	# of Reps	Weight	# of Reps
Barbell Standing Military Press Set 1				
Barbell Standing Military Press Set 2				
Barbell Standing Military Press Set 3				
Barbell Standing Military Press Set 4				
Neutral Grip Overhead Dumbbell Press Set 1				
Neutral Grip Overhead Dumbbell Press Set 2				
Neutral Grip Overhead Dumbbell Press Set 3				
Dumbbell Lateral Raise Set 1				
Dumbbell Lateral Raise Set 2				
Dumbbell Lateral Raise Set 3				
Dumbbell Shrugs Set 1				
Dumbbell Shrugs Set 2				
Dumbbell Shrugs Set 3				
Cable Face Pulls Set 1				
Cable Face Pulls Set 2				
Cable Face Pulls Set 3				
Link to Barbell Standing Military Press Guide: https://www.youtube.com/watch?v=L0CR9_-f82k				

My Personal Workout Regime

Below I have set out for you my personal workout regime at the time of writing this book. There are so many different workout plans out there and it can be hard to decide which to choose. The important thing is to find something that works for you. This workout plan works for me and it could possibly work for you too.

I have been using this plan, which I developed myself, for eight weeks now and I have noticed some good results. It's only a 4 day a week plan and on my off days I try to do some stretching and light cardio. For each set I try to stick to between 10-12 reps. As soon as I get to 12 reps in a specific exercise I move up the weight. Give it a shot, you may like it, but be warned Day 2 is a killer.

Day 1 – Chest, Triceps, and Shoulders				
	Week 1		Week 2	
Exercise	Weight	# of Reps	Weight	# of Reps
Flat Dumbbell Bench Press Set 1				
Flat Dumbbell Bench Press Set 2				
Incline Dumbbell Bench Press Set 1				
Incline Dumbbell Bench Press Set 2				
Decline Barbell Bench Press Set 1				
Decline Barbell Bench Press Set 2				
Tricep Skull Crushers Set 1				
Tricep Skull Crushers Set 2				
Tricep Skull Crushers Set 3				
Tricep Cable Pull Down Set 1				
Tricep Cable Pull Down Set 2				
Tricep Cable Pull Down Set 3				
Arnold Press Set 1				
Arnold Press Set 2				
Arnold Press Set 3				
Arnold Press Set 4				
Rear Deltoid Fly Set 1				
Rear Deltoid Fly Set 2				

Day 2 – Back, Legs, and Abs				
	Week 1		Week 2	
Exercise	Weight	# of Reps	Weight	# of Reps
Deadlift Set 1				
Deadlift Set 2				
Deadlift Set 3				
Deadlift Set 4				
Pull Ups Set 1				
Pull Ups Set 2				
Dumbbell Goblet Squat Set 1				
Dumbbell Goblet Squat Set 2				
Dumbbell Goblet Squat Set 3				
Weighted Lunges Set 1				
Weighted Lunges Set 2				
Weighted Lunges Set 3				
Weighted Decline Sit Ups Set 1				
Weighted Decline Sit Ups Set 2				
Weighted Decline Sit Ups Set 3				
Weighted Decline Sit Ups Set 4				
Leg Raises Set 1				
Leg Raises Set 2				

Weight Training For Dumbbells

Day 3 – Shoulders, Chest, and Triceps				
	Week 1		Week 2	
Exercise	Weight	# of Reps	Weight	# of Reps
Military Press Set 1				
Military Press Set 2				
Military Press Set 3				
Military Press Set 4				
Dumbbell Lateral Raise Set 1				
Dumbbell Lateral Raise Set 2				
Flat Dumbbell Bench Press Set 1				
Flat Dumbbell Bench Press Set 2				
Incline Dumbbell Bench Press Set 1				
Incline Dumbbell Bench Press Set 2				
Decline Barbell Bench Press Set 1				
Decline Barbell Bench Press Set 2				
Neutral Grip Dumbbell Bench Press Set 1				
Neutral Grip Dumbbell Bench Press Set 2				
Neutral Grip Dumbbell Bench Press Set 3				
Tricep Skull Crushers Set 1				
Tricep Skull Crushers Set 2				
Tricep Skull Crushers Set 3				

Day 4 – Legs, Back, and Biceps				
	Week 1		Week 2	
Exercise	Weight	# of Reps	Weight	# of Reps
Squats Set 1				
Squats Set 2				
Squats Set 3				
Squats Set 4				
Weighted Calf Raises Set 1				
Weighted Calf Raises Set 2				
Seated Row Set 1				
Seated Row Set 2				
Seated Row Set 3				
Pull Ups Set 1				
Pull Ups Set 2				
Pull Ups Set 3				
Dumbbell Bicep Curls Set 1				
Dumbbell Bicep Curls Set 2				
Reverse Barbell Curl Set 1				
Reverse Barbell Curl Set 2				
Dumbbell Hammer Curl Set 1				
Dumbbell Hammer Curl Set 2				

Conclusion

Everyone's journey is going to be different and we are all going to take different paths. With a basic understanding of how weightlifting works you are now better off than half the people in the gym. Hopefully by reading this book you will realize the importance of proper nutrition, proper form, keeping track of your progress, and being consistent in the gym.

In the end I will be glad to hear that my experience has taught you and has saved you time or money. I'm so lucky to be able to help people and give them advice based on my experience. I would like to thank YOU the reader for supporting me and allowing me to teach you the basics.

Remember what I've taught you, and be sure to apply the information I have given you to your meals, workouts, and life. I wish you all the best and hope you all have a fantastic ride on your weightlifting journey.

God Bless,

Liam McEachen, B.Bus.